# How To Get Rid Of Back Pain

## 330 Great Tips To Treat And Cure Back Pain

## ADAM COLTON

Published by BizMove
www.bizmove.com

# Table of Contents


1  Back Pain  Fact Sheet                                              5

2  330 Great Tips To Treat And Cure Back                             19
   Pain

# 1. Back Pain Fact Sheet

Back pain is one of the most common medical problems in the U.S. It can range from a dull, constant ache to a sudden, sharp pain that puts you out of action. Sometimes it can come on suddenly—from an accident, a fall, or lifting something heavy. In other cases, it can develop slowly due to age-related changes to the spine.

## Points To Remember About Back Pain

- Back pain is one of the most common medical problems in the U.S.
- Acute pain is the most common type of back pain and lasts no longer than 6 weeks. Chronic pain can come on quickly or slowly and lasts a long time, generally longer than 3 months.
- Anyone can have back pain, but some things increase the risk.
- Back pain is a symptom of a medical condition. It can get better even if you do not know the cause.
- Treatment for back pain generally depends on how long your pain lasts.
- Exercise, proper diet, and hot and cold packs can help you live better with back pain.

## Who Gets

Although anyone can have back pain, a number of factors increase your risk. They include:

- **Age**: Back pain becomes more common with age, with the first attack typically between ages 30 and 40.
- **Fitness level**: Back pain is more common among people who are not physically fit. For example, weak back and stomach muscles may not properly support the spine. Back pain is also more likely if you exercise a lot after being inactive for a while.
- **Diet**: A diet high in calories and fat, combined with an inactive lifestyle, can lead to obesity. This can put stress on the back.
- **Heredity**: Genetics play a role in some disorders that cause back pain.
- **Race**: African American women are more likely than white women to develop spondylolisthesis, a condition in which bones in the lower spine slip out of place.
- **Other diseases**: Back pain may be caused or worsened by some diseases, such as certain types of arthritis and cancers that spread to the spine.
- **Job-related risk factors**: Jobs that requires heavy lifting, pushing, pulling, or twisting can injure the back. A desk job may also play a role,

especially if you have poor posture or sit all day in an uncomfortable chair.

- **Cigarette smoking**: Although smoking may not directly cause back pain, it increases your risk of developing low back pain and sciatica, which is back pain that travels to the hip and/or leg. Smoking can also slow healing from back injuries or surgeries.

## Types

- **Acute pain** is pain that hits you suddenly after an accident, a fall, or lifting something heavy. Acute pain is the most common type of back pain and lasts no longer than six weeks.
- **Chronic pain** may come on either quickly or slowly and lasts a long time, generally longer than three months. This type of back pain is much less common.

## Causes

Back pain can be caused by many different things, including:

- **Mechanical problems** in the way your spine moves or the way you feel when you move your spine in certain ways. Mechanical causes of back pain include break-down of the disks between the bones of the spine, ruptured disks, spasms, and muscle tension.

- **Injuries** such as sprains and fractures can cause either short-lived or chronic pain. Sprains are tears in the ligaments that support the spine, and they can occur from twisting or lifting improperly. Fractured vertebrae are often the result of osteoporosis. Less commonly, back pain may be caused by more severe injuries that result from accidents or falls.
- **Medical conditions** can cause or contribute to back pain. They include:
    - *Scoliosis*, curving of the spine that does not usually cause pain until middle age.
    - *Spondylolisthesis*, where a bone in the spine slips out of place.
    - Various forms of *arthritis*.
    - *Spinal stenosis*, a narrowing of the spinal column that puts pressure on the spinal cord and nerves.
    - *Osteoporosis*, which can lead to painful fractures of the vertebrae.
    - *Pregnancy*.
    - *Kidney stones* or infections.
    - *Endometriosis*, which is the buildup of uterine tissue in places outside the uterus.
    - *Fibromyalgia*, a condition of widespread muscle pain and fatigue.

- o *Infections* can cause pain when they involve the bones of the spine or the disks between these bones.
- o *Tumors* can cause back pain in rare cases. Tumors may appear in the back or be the result of cancer that has spread from other parts of the body.
- **Stress** can worsen pain by causing back muscles to become tense and painful.

## Treatment

Treatment for back pain generally depends on how long your pain lasts:

- **Acute (short-term) back pain** usually gets better on its own. Exercises or surgery are usually not recommended for acute back pain. There are some things you may try while you wait for your pain to get better:
  - o Acetaminophen, aspirin, or ibuprofen will help ease the pain.
  - o Get up and move around to ease stiffness, relieve pain, and have you back doing your regular activities sooner.
- **Chronic (long-term) back pain** is typically treated with nonsurgical options before surgery is recommended.
  - o *Nonsurgical Treatments*:

- <u>Hot or cold packs</u> can be soothing to constantly sore, stiff backs.
- <u>Exercise</u> can help ease chronic pain and may reduce the risk of it returning. Check with your doctor before starting a new exercise routine.
- <u>Medications</u> to treat chronic back pain are available over the counter or by prescription.
  - Pain relievers that are taken by mouth or applied to the skin. Examples include acetaminophen and aspirin.
  - Nonsteroidal anti-inflammatory drugs (NSAIDs) relieve pain and inflammation. Examples include ibuprofen, ketoprofen, and naproxen sodium.
  - Muscle relaxants and some antidepressants may be prescribed for some types of chronic back pain.
  - Your doctor may suggest steroid or numbing shots to lessen your pain.
- <u>Traction</u> involves using pulleys and weights to stretch the back, which may allow a bulging disk to slip back

into place. Your pain may be relieved while in traction, although pain returns once you aren't in traction.

- <u>Behavioral modification</u> teaches you to:
    - Move your body properly while you do daily activities, especially those involving heavy lifting, pushing, or pulling.
    - Practice healthy habits, such as exercise, relaxation, regular sleep, proper diet, and quitting smoking.
- <u>Complementary and alternative treatments</u> are an option when medications and other therapies do not relieve pain. Examples include:
    - *Manipulation.* Professionals use their hands to adjust or massage the spine or nearby tissues.
    - *Transcutaneous electrical nerve stimulation* (TENS). A small box over the painful area sends mild electrical pulses to nerves. TENS treatments are not always effective for reducing pain.

- *Acupuncture.* This Chinese practice uses thin needles to relieve pain and restore health. Acupuncture may be effective when used as a part of a comprehensive treatment plan for low back pain.
- *Acupressure.* A therapist applies pressure to certain places in the body to relieve pain. Acupressure has not been well studied for back pain.

- *Surgical treatments* may be necessary in some cases, including:
  - **Herniated (ruptured) disks** are when one or more of the disks that cushion the bones of the spine are damaged. The jelly-like center of the disk leaks, causing pain. Common surgeries include:
    - *Laminectomy/diskectomy*, which removes a portion of spinal bone as well as the damaged disk.
    - *Microdiskectomy*, which removes a damaged disk but through a smaller incision compared to laminectomy/diskectomy.

- *Laser surgery* uses a needle that produces bursts of laser energy to reduce the size of the damaged disk. This relieves pressure on the nerves. The usefulness of this procedure is still being debated.
- **Spinal stenosis**, a narrowing of the spinal column that puts pressure on the spinal cord and nerves, is treated by laminectomy. This is a major surgery that opens up the spinal column. A short hospital stay and physical therapy will be required after the surgery.
- **Spondylolisthesis**, where one or more bones in the spine slip out of place. This is treated by laminectomy and spinal fusion, which joins two of the spinal bones together so that they don't move.
- **Vertebral fractures** caused by injury to the bones in the spine or by osteoporosis. This is treated by:
  - *Vertebroplasty* involves injecting a cement-like mixture into the fractured bone to relieve pain and stabilize the spine.

- *Kyphoplasty* relieves pain and stabilizes the spine following fractures caused by osteoporosis. Doctors insert a balloon-device to help restore the height and shape of the spine and then inject a cement-like mixture to repair the fractured bone.

- **Degenerative disk disease**, or damage to the spine's disks as a person gets older. This can be treated by:
  - *Intradiskal electrothermal therapy (IDET)* is one of the least invasive therapies for low back pain. Doctors insert a heating wire into the damaged disk and pass an electrical current through the wire to strengthen the fibers that hold the disk together. The effectiveness of IDET is not clear.
  - *Spinal fusion*, which involves removing and fusing the damaged disk to help with the pain.

- *Disk replacement* replaces the damaged disk with a synthetic one.

Back pain is a symptom of a medical condition, not a diagnosis itself. In rare cases, back pain is caused by a tumor, an infection, or a nerve root problem called cauda equina syndrome. In these cases, surgery is needed right away to ease the pain and prevent more problems.

You probably don't need to see your doctor for back pain, unless you have:

- Numbness and tingling.
- Severe back pain that does not improve with medication.
- Back pain after a fall or injury.
- Back pain along with:
    - Trouble urinating.
    - Weakness, pain, or numbness in your legs.
    - Fever.
    - Weight loss that you didn't intend.

## Who Treats

Many different types of doctors treat back pain:

- Family or primary care doctors (usually seen first).
- Doctors who specialize in disorders of the nerves, muscles, or skeleton.

## Living With

There are a few things you can do to help you live with back pain:

- Hot or cold packs can be soothing to constantly sore, stiff backs. Heat dilates the blood vessels to increase blood supply to the back and reduce muscle spasms. Cold may reduce inflammation and numb deep pain.
- Exercise can help ease chronic pain and may reduce the risk of it returning. Check with your doctor before starting a new exercise routine, which may include the following:
  - *Flexion exercises* have you bending forward to reduce pressure on the nerves, stretch the back and hip muscles, and strengthen the stomach and buttock muscles.
  - *Extension* involve bending backward, such as lying on your stomach while you lift your leg or raise your trunk. These exercises may reduce pain that spreads from one place and develop muscles that support the spine.

- *Stretching* improves the extension of muscles and other soft tissues of the back. These exercises can reduce back stiffness and improve range of motion.
- *Aerobic exercise* gets your heart pumping faster and include brisk walking, jogging, and swimming. Avoid exercise that requires twisting, bending forward quickly, such as aerobic dancing and rowing. Avoid high-impact activities if you have disk disease.

## Prevention

Work with your doctor to develop a plan to help prevent many types of back pain. The plan should include:

- Regular exercise that keeps your back muscles strong. Exercises that increase balance and strength can decrease your risk of falling and injuring your back or breaking bones. Exercises such as tai chi and yoga—or any weight-bearing exercise that challenges your balance—are good ones to try.
- Eating a healthy diet that includes enough calcium and vitamin D, nutrients that keep your spine strong. A healthy diet also helps in

controlling weight to avoid putting unnecessary and injury-causing stress and strain on your back.

- Practicing good posture, supporting your back properly, and avoiding heavy lifting when possible.

# 2. 330 Great Tips To Treat And Cure Back Pain

Back pain is not only painful, but can definitely be debilitating. The best way to deal with your back pain involves getting involved in your diagnosis, understanding back pain, and learning the best methods for you individually. These back pain tips will give you a great deal of helping in finding your way toward pain relief.

1.  If your back pain gets to be too debilitating, consider seeking professional help. If you have insurance, there is a good chance it might cover a few sessions. Trained physical therapists can give you helpful advice and help you to develop an exercise regimen that will work to strengthen your back.

2.  Remain as active as possible during a bout of back pain, as it has been shown that activity is more helpful to recovery than lying in bed. Try to carry out normal activities, within reason, as studies have shown that this leads to a more rapid recovery than bed rest or back-specific exercise.

3. Apply topical pain relievers to help relieve back pain. Various creams, oils, gels and medicated patches are available that can be applied to the area of the back that hurts in order to offer pain relief. Many can be found over the counter, but some can only be obtained from a medical practitioner or by prescription.

4. When dealing with back problems, it is best to use cold instead of heat to soothe pain. Some people might not have much luck with heating pads and hot compresses. Experts have found that cold to soothe can work just as well. It might not be as comfortable, but it can be effective in relieving pain. You might want to give it a shot and see what works best for you.

5. Some people have to work and stand for long hours at a time. If you must do this, then make sure you try and stand tall and straight. Try and allow your legs to rest too from time to time if possible, perhaps on a stool or bench if you are allowed to do that.

6. Maintain proper posture at all times to alleviate back pain. Many adults have pain from being hunched over and not even realizing it. When you are sitting or standing, make sure that your

back is extremely straight. It might feel uncomfortable at first. Although your body will get used to it, and your back will thank you later.

7. Lower back pain is the main form of back pain, and it is the 2nd most common reason for people going to see a doctor. It may be that your daily routine is contributing to your back pain, so a few simple changes can provide some relief. Lower back pains appear very easily, which is why you should do your best to prevent it.

8. Eating a healthy diet not only helps keep your weight at a good level, but also a balanced healthy diet with plenty of Vitamin D keeps your bones strong which means your back stays strong. A balanced diet is important for every aspect of health, so not surprisingly, it is no different with your back health.

9. One area of your life that can be affected by chronic back pain is your sex life. If left covered up, you are not allowing your partner to be understanding of your back pain. Your partner may think another reason is putting a strain on you guys' sex life. Therefore, it is imperative to be open and honest and look for ways for your back pain not to disrupt your sex life.

10. Unless you have recently had back surgery, it is important that you try to avoid wearing back braces. There is no medical evidence proving that it helps back conditions or pain. In fact, recent studies suggest that it may aggravate certain back conditions and even cause the pain to worsen.

11. In order to prevent upper back pain, be sure that your arms are at a comfortable level when using the computer. Many back strains are caused by people extending and raising their arms too high or too low when they have to use the computer for prolonged periods of time.

12. A great way to fight against back pain is to actually fight against your stress levels. Having high levels of stress can easily trigger a back spasm or general back pain. Even if it's psychosomatic, the pain is still real enough, so remember to try to get rid of your stress in order to get rid of back pain.

13. If you want to eliminate back pain, you should try to stay properly hydrated. Drinking plenty of water is great for your overall health, but it is especially good for your muscle health. Muscles are essentially water and protein, and once you

start to become dehydrated. Your muscles can easily spasm.

14. Many people know that exercise and proper posture can help relieve their back pain, but did you know that sometimes all you actually need to do is to de-stress? You may think your back pain is causing your stress, but actually it might be your stress causing your pain.

15. One good way to avoid back pain is to avoid situations that cause back spasms. These triggers include lack of sleep, caffeine, dehydration, low sodium, anxiety, and stress. When you do have a back spasm, rest with a hot pack on your back to help the pain subside.

16. As your teacher may have told you when you were young, you shouldn't have bad posture, so work to keep the right posture if you want to help ease your back pain. Always strive to keep your back straight, your shoulders squared, and your head high. This is the body's natural position.

17. Use over the counter pain relievers, such as ibuprofen and acetaminophen, to help relieve back pain. Taking oral pain medications can allow you to function somewhat normally when

you are suffering from a bout of back pain. Be sure to follow the instructions on the package for best results.

18. You can prevent unnecessary back injuries even without a brace. To reduce the amount of strain your back absorbs, always stand with your feet shoulder width apart and bend and lift from your knees instead of from your back. Centering heavy items prior to lifting them also helps to prevent strain.

19. Always take time to stretch, regardless of whether you will encounter strenuous activity. If you stretch, you are giving your back more preparation for the day ahead, without which you could be allowing yourself to experience pain and even injuries. Even if you aren't planning a stressful day, you want to make sure that you are stretching sufficiently to loosen those muscles in the back that are used so often.

20. Make sure you're maintaining a proper weight. If you're overweight, particularly if that weight is in your upper body, you'll be putting a lot more pressure on your back and spine. By keeping an optimum weight, you'll make sure you're not putting too much stress on your back and spine.

21. Strengthening your muscles is as important to healing from a back injury as it is to preventing future injury. That said, people already experiencing back pain should not engage in exercises that put undue strain on their injured muscles. For that reason, walking briskly every day is the best way to work through injuries while also working all the muscles in your body to prevent future injuries.

22. To help relieve back pain resulting from strained or injured back muscles, give your back plenty of rest. Strained back muscles need rest and recovery, which speeds up the healing process. Try lying on your back or on your side, whichever is most comfortable for you. Keep your spine properly aligned in its normal position. Some people find that lying on firm surfaces, like a firm mattress or a carpeted floor, helps immensely.

23. Make sure you watch your posture at all times, whether standing or sitting. Poor posture leads to back problems. You should sit up in your chair at all times, and arm rests are important on chairs if possible to allow your back the support it needs. Extended use of a chair without arm rests can really put a strain on the back.

24. Try not to stand for long periods of time. Doing this can cause a back injury because of all the strain that you are putting your body through. If you have a job that causes you to be on your feet all day, make sure to sit on your breaks, and when you get home you rest for a little.

25. No matter what the reason, if you suffer from back pain and you have to bend over, be sure to do so with your knees and not your back. Many people suffer from back strains or pains because they bend over using their back, which puts too much pressure on the spine.

26. Quitting smoking can help to ease back pain. People who smoke, especially heavy smokers, do not have as much blood flow to the spine as those who don't smoke. Without a sufficient amount of blood flow to the spine, your back will hurt.

27. Many people confuse resting and relaxation with each other. Resting is necessary to help prevent back pain, but too much rest can actually hinder it. Once you rest, you must begin to relax or else you are not fully benefiting from your time of rest. Relaxing is realizing your position and allowing your body to surrender to relaxation.

28. If you suffer from chronic back pain, getting a simple massage can help to eliminate the pain and muscle cramping. Whether you're visiting a massage therapist or just relaxing in one of those massaging chairs, receiving a massage can help to loosen the muscles and subsequently relieve the pain of a back ache.

29. A lot of people who do not sleep on a regular schedule experience back pain, so try to get at least seven hours of sleep per night on a regular schedule. Staying awake and on your feet for prolonged hours puts a lot of stress on your back and can ultimately result in moderate to severe pain. Sleeping will help decrease this.

30. As a back pain sufferer, a little bit of pain may actually make you feel better, so do not be afraid to exercise. The reason you feel pain is because the muscles are sore and stiff. If you can work through this and loosen the muscles up, you can do light exercise and help to get rid of the pain.

31. If you like to wear high heels but experience back pain, the answer is simple; take the heels off and go with regular shoes. Standing on your toes is a very unnatural posture for your spine. Over time, this can cause damage to not only your

muscles but also the discs in your back. Save the high heels for very special occasions.

32. If your back pain gets to be too debilitating, consider seeking professional help. If you have insurance, there is a good chance it might cover a few sessions. Trained physical therapists can give you helpful advice and help you to develop an exercise regimen that will work to strengthen your back.

33. To aid your body in healing from painful back injuries, invest in a firm mattress. Many people mistakenly believe that a soft mattress will be more comforting to their injured back. In truth, a soft mattress will not help you to maintain your posture through the night while a firm mattress gives your back the support it needs to repair itself.

34. Make sure you drink enough water. The human body is primarily water, including our muscles and the discs in our spines. Getting enough water helps increase the size of the intervertebral discs, which will keep your spine flexible and reduce your back pain. You really can't drink too much water.

35. Many people try to pick up things that are a good distance away from them because they are trying to rush. People often take shortcuts and they do this daily. Avoid straining your back by moving closer to objects before lifting them and follow the proper instructions for safe lifting.

36. If you suffer from issues with the cartilage in your spine, you can avoid pain by avoiding sitting for long periods of time. Sitting compresses the disks in your spine, because it causes your abdomen to press backwards. Try reclining, or using a lumbar cushion if you must sit, and take frequent breaks to stand up.

37. Keeping your back, pain free, is usually a couple of fairly simple techniques. If you are hurting in a certain spot try massaging the muscle group around that particular area. Do a few stretches and apply a heating pad. Some people also find it helpful to use a vibrating chair like the ones at the mall.

38. Taking a pillow with you on long drives can help to relieve back pain. By placing a soft pillow between the small of your back and the seat of the automobile, you are creating a cushioned support that will help you maintain proper

posture when driving those long hours and thus help to decrease back pain.

39. Being overweight is one of the biggest causes of back pain in the world, so always attempt to maintain a healthy weight if you're fighting back pain. You will find as an overweight individual that as you begin to lose the weight, your back pain will lessen. The goal should be to keep fighting to lose the weight.

40. If your back pain does not improve or continues to get worse, you may want to look into a chiropractor. They can take X-rays and discuss potential treatments with you based off of the findings. Soon enough, with gentle adjustments, your pain will ease.

41. There can be many causes for back pain and you will want to be sure to identify what is causing the pain before you try to do anything to resolve it. Try changing up some minor things in your life to see if these have any effect on your pain.

42. Being overweight can lead to back problems. Having to carry around extra weight puts a lot of strain on the back. If you do need to lose a couple of pounds to help your back feel better,

set small goals for yourself so that you can achieve success often.

43. Find ways to make your daily work activities more active! Invest in a telephone headset so you can walk around your office during a conference call. Walk to someone's office instead of picking up the phone. These habit changes will get you out of your chair and relieve a lot of back pain in the process.

44. If your job involves standing still for long periods of time, this can be a major cause of back strain. One method of reducing this strain is to have a prop like a box or small footstool to alternately put your foot on. This relaxes some muscles and stretches the back.

45. Get a hot tub. In addition to the many health benefits that spas provide, such as better circulation and a general feeling of relaxation, spas can also soothe back pain. Get a personal spa and have a nice bubbly soak every day and you'll notice that your back feels much better.

46. Medical science has devised specific exercises for back pain that target strengthening bones and muscles to alleviate the problem! Ask your doctor or go on line for a list and diagrams of

some very helpful and simple exercises you can do every morning that will help your body become stronger and more capable of sustaining the everyday stress and strain that takes such a toll on your back!

47. When you have lower back pain, try using an exercise ball to provide relief. Doing appropriate exercises on the ball will help you develop flexibility and increase the tone of your lower back muscles. As your back muscles become stronger, they will give your lower back better support, thus reducing your pain.

48. Stop when your back hurts. People who suffer with chronic back pain sometimes try to work through the pain or to keep going when their back hurts. This can make your back pain worse and increase any damage you've already done. Always take the opportunity to rest for a while so that you don't hurt your back further.

49. Use over the counter pain relievers, such as ibuprofen and acetaminophen, to help relieve back pain. Taking oral pain medications can allow you to function somewhat normally when you are suffering from a bout of back pain. Be sure to follow the instructions on the package for best results.

50. When dealing with back problems, it is best to use cold instead of heat to soothe pain. Some people might not have much luck with heating pads and hot compresses. Experts have found that cold to soothe can work just as well. It might not be as comfortable, but it can be effective in relieving pain. You might want to give it a shot and see what works best for you.

51. Start eating in a healthy way and drink a lot of water, about eight to ten cups a day. There are many things that a nutritious diet can do for you, and helping to prevent back pain is one of them. Less pressure will be applied to your back if you lose weight, and certain nutrients are essential for a generally healthy body and good blood circulation.

52. In order to avoid back pain, avoid sitting for extended periods of time. Sitting is bad for your back. If you must sit at a desk all day, get up every so often and stretch or walk around. Likewise, if you spend a lot of time in the car, take frequent breaks so that you can stretch your legs.

53. Some people have to work and stand for long hours at a time. If you must do this, then make

sure you try and stand tall and straight. Try and allow your legs to rest too from time to time if possible, perhaps on a stool or bench if you are allowed to do that.

54. To prevent getting back pain, you need to make sure that you exercise on a regular basis. This will help increase and strengthen the muscles in your back. You just need to be careful that you are not lifting weights that are too heavy and that you are not doing anything else that could actually cause an injury.

55. Try not to stand for long periods of time. Doing this can cause a back injury because of all the strain that you are putting your body through. If you have a job that causes you to be on your feet all day, make sure to sit on your breaks, and when you get home you rest for a little.

56. It may seem to go against common sense, but those with back injuries and pain should exercise often. People dealing with back pain usually think that activity will worsen their pain, but the opposite is true. Tight muscles in your back can contribute to or even cause back pain. Exercising can help stretch your back muscles and reduce pain.

57. If you suffer from back pain, remember to stay aware of your posture when sitting down. This is especially important for those who sit in an office chair all day because slumping over your desk can do a number on your spine. Remember to have the soles of your feet flat on the ground and your back as straight and upright as possible.

58. Undoubtedly, one of the best possible methods to relieve back pain is to exercise regularly. You do not have to become a cardio enthusiast or a quasi weight-lifter, but exercising every day will work wonders in relieving back pain associated with cramping muscles. The physical activity can really help to get rid of the pain.

59. Many people know that exercise and proper posture can help relieve their back pain, but did you know that sometimes all you actually need to do is to de-stress? You may think your back pain is causing your stress, but actually it might be your stress causing your pain.

60. To address back pain, take up yoga. Even if you are in poor physical condition, you can begin with some simple, easy positions that will help stretch your back muscles and loosen tension. By strengthening and lengthening the muscles of the

back and releasing tension in the spine, you will eliminate your back pain.

61. A good time for stretching is when the muscles have not yet cooled down. After completing and exercise session, be sure to stretch during your cool-down time.

62. Visit your local natural foods or holistic store to see if they offer any back pain remedies. There are many products and remedies on the market today, and it is really more effective to simply shop around and see what's available than to try to list them all. Just ask an employee what remedies they have for back pain.

63. Getting into Pilates or yoga is a great way in which you can work to alleviate or even permanently eliminate back pain. Yoga and Pilates focuses more on stretching, elongating and strengthening the muscles, which is perfect for your back and can easily help to eliminate some of your pain.

64. Even children can experience a lot of back pain, so make sure that your kids aren't carrying heavy loads in their backpacks. This tip also goes for hikers and campers out there who lug around

heavy luggage on their backs. Lighten your load to assist in eliminating your back pain.

65. Good posture is one of the most vital components to a healthy back! Back pain can be an awful obstacle in our daily lives and even give us trouble while we try to sleep! One of the best things you can do for your back is maintain proper posture while walking or standing and most definitely while you are sitting so keep your spine straight and avoid any forward leaning.

66. If your back pain gets to be too debilitating, consider seeking professional help. If you have insurance, there is a good chance it might cover a few sessions. Trained physical therapists can give you helpful advice and help you to develop an exercise regimen that will work to strengthen your back.

67. Use ice to help alleviate back pain, as it can reduce swelling and inflammation from injuries that cause back pain. Apply the ice to the affected area two or three times per day for 10 to 20 minutes, and this may help you feel better. An ice pack or a bag of frozen vegetables can be used for this purpose.

68. It's simple to protect your back when you are spending hours sitting at a desk. Just take a break to walk around. You can stretch your back muscles by simply standing up and doing a few leg stretches, or walking. This helps to avoid injuries related to compression of the lumbar discs.

69. Some people have to work and stand for long hours at a time. If you must do this, then make sure you try and stand tall and straight. Try and allow your legs to rest too from time to time if possible, perhaps on a stool or bench if you are allowed to do that.

70. How many times have you seen a woman carrying a heavy purse on one shoulder? How many times have you seen a student carrying his or her backpack on one shoulder? You should always make heavy loads proportionate, and also make sure to limit the amount of time you have to carry them on a consistent basis.

71. Make sure that your home and work environment is set up safely. You do not want to have a bunch of stuff on the floor that you could easily trip on and seriously hurt your back. Take a couple minutes each day and make sure that your house is picked-up.

72. In order to heal your back, you must remove yourself from the source of pain. Once removed, then find yourself a place to rest. Whether it be a comfortable chair, recliner or even a place to lay down. Find a position that offers you the most support to relieve your back tension.

73. Many women suffer from back pain during pregnancy. A growing baby changes your center of gravity and causes you to lean back to counteract this, causing pain in the lower back. The best remedy for this is good posture. Sit straight and keep your shoulders back. Sit in a comfortable chair and relax. Baby your back while you wait for baby!

74. Seek the Hatha Yoga Sun Salutation online for a series of gentle, easy stretches that you can perform every morning and every night to strengthen your back and lengthen your spine. Performing this gentle series of exercises for fifteen minutes, twice a day can work wonders to eliminate your back pain.

75. Spending a lot of time behind the wheel or in the passenger seat is a big reason so many people deal with back pain in this automobile age. While driving, take care to adjust your seat in relation to

the steering wheel, as well as the pedals of your car. You need to be able to reach these without having to stretch your back.

76. You should know that the proper sleep can help you to get rid of back pain, but more important is the actually position in which you're sleeping. Make sure that you're not tossing and turning and make sure that your body is aligned properly while you're sleeping. A great pillow and comfortable mattress go a long way to helping you keep back pain at bay.

77. Be sure to spend about five minutes stretching your muscles, while they are still warm, before and after a workout to avoid straining back muscles. When you have finished exercising, ensure you also stretch.

78. Visit health food stores and other places that sell herbal remedies and other alternative medications for back pain. The list of natural remedies is long and every store sells something different. Chiropractic care, acupuncture and massages are alternative remedies for relieving back pain.

79. Doing the simple things can help you alleviate back pain, like simply taking your time when you

stand up or get out of bed. Sudden movements and jerking motions can jar the muscles and even cause discs to slip and slide around. Be cognizant of your movements and take a little time when getting up.

80. Sleeping on the stomach is not an option, and if you sleep on your back, it can strain it. Your weight will be more evenly distributed if you learn to enjoy sleeping on your side.

81. A foot stool at your desk can help your back to relax if you find yourself sitting for long periods of time; this goes a long way towards relieving back pain. As soon as you feel back pain, you should elevate your feet a bit. The elevation of your feet should help stop pain before it gets worse.

82. Developing a B12 deficiency can drain your energy and wreak havoc on your muscles, and this also means you're at a much higher risk of severe back pain. So it's important that you keep up with your intake of B vitamins. Try vitamin supplements and various meat sources to get the sufficient amount of B12.

83. Don't ignore the pain. If you know a particular activity is going to exacerbate your pain, then

don't do that activity. Ignoring it will not make it go away faster. In fact, pushing through the pain will probably result in further injury, making the pain last even longer.

84. Consider switching your most commonly used chair into an ergonomic chair. There are several ergonomically designed chairs these days that are made just for those that are sitting at a desk or sitting up all day. These chairs promote better positioning within the chair, thus offering a greater amount of comfort and less stress on your back.

85. Try not to stand for long periods of time. Doing this can cause a back injury because of all the strain that you are putting your body through. If you have a job that causes you to be on your feet all day, make sure to sit on your breaks, and when you get home you rest for a little.

86. Several different types of medications exist that can help with back pain. Again, it is important that you make sure to consult your doctor before making any decisions. Many times OTC medication can suffice, but other times you need a prescription, like for painkillers.

87. Although many people believe otherwise, people who have back pain must exercise frequently. Many of those afflicted by back pain believe that exercising will make their pain worse, but that simply is not always the case. When the back muscles are stretched, it often helps alleviate back pain.

88. Unless you have recently had back surgery, it is important that you try to avoid wearing back braces. There is no medical evidence proving that it helps back conditions or pain. In fact, recent studies suggest that it may aggravate certain back conditions and even cause the pain to worsen.

89. When working at your desk or computer, make sure you sit in the proper posture or purchase an ergonomic chair. Be sure to get up and walk around and loosen your muscles. It is easier to keep them from getting cramped rather than trying to get out the cramps in your back.

90. A lot of back pain sufferers, find that lying on their stomachs can help to relieve the pain. Most lower back pain comes from strain and stress, and lying on the back can actually intensify this due to the muscle tension. Lying on your

stomach, however, can relax these muscles and relieve the pain.

91. Some living a sedentary lifestyle will experience chronic bouts of back pain, so it's always a great idea to ensure that you're getting up and moving around for at least 30 minutes of the day. Experiencing back pain while sitting and then going to lie down can create a cycle that results in severe pain at frequent intervals.

92. If you have chronic back pain and cannot figure out how to get rid of it, perhaps a new chair is in order, like a recliner or something softer than what you're sitting on now. A lot of people think that firm support is a must, but that's more to prevent pain. If you need to relieve it, go with something soft.

93. While back pain is certainly more commonly found in the elderly this does not indicate that younger people will not experience it. If you are not living an active lifestyle you can have back pain at a very young age. This is also true for people who play heavy sports.

94. Stomach and back sleeping are both out of the question if your belly is large sized, in particular

if there is a child in there. Side sleeping distributes weight evenly.

95. People with anxiety issues can become tense, this can lead to muscle strains and spasms and then lead to back pain. Work on various ways to overcome your anxiety with relaxation techniques and as an added bonus you can get rid of back pain.

96. If you're thinking about purchasing anything at all to assist with your back pain, look in to purchasing an ergonomic chair. These types of chairs are specifically designed for your back and will provide full support that you can rely on. You can keep proper posture while sitting in these chairs and alleviate and possibly even eliminate your pain.

97. If you're riding in the car for long periods, try putting a towel in the arch of your back for extra support. Also, make sure to move your seat a little forward or back every once in a while so that your spine has a chance to move and doesn't get stiff.

98. Get more vitamin D. Vitamin D has been shown to cause chronic back pain in some cases, but getting more of this important vitamin is an

easy thing to do. Have some milk and spend time outside to get the most vitamin D you can. Most people are vitamin D deficient and don't know that, so make sure to talk to your doctor about checking your blood to be sure.

99. Stair climbing is a good exercise to strengthen the back muscles and help relieve back pain. When stair climbing, either with a machine or on actual stairs, make sure to keep your posture good, as if you were balancing a book on your head. Slumping over can hurt your back more.

100.   Taking a warm bath can help to relieve back pain. Warmth loosens tight muscles and helps you to relax. Sitting in a bath has relaxing properties all its own. Enjoy the bath for as long as you are comfortable and keep the water warm, but not too hot, to avoid burning your sensitive skin.

101.   To help prevent or alleviate back pain, try walking each day. Research has indicated that walking helps relieve back pain, whereas doing specific exercises meant to alleviate back pain may actually make the pain worse. Although your back may hurt, it is important to walk briskly for three hours per week to obtain relief.

102.    It may take a day or more to get an appointment to treat a serious back injury, and in that time many people have a hard time sitting or lying comfortably. For many sufferers, it is comfortable to lay flat on their back with there knees bent, no matter what the injury is. This position reduces tension in the tendons and muscles which start in the back and continue through the legs.

103.    Be careful when lifting. Always use proper posture when lifting. Lift from the knees. Lifting heavy object improperly can really do quite a number on your back. To avoid causing potentially permanent damage, use caution. If the object is too heavy to lift request assistance or use a moving dolly.

104.    If you read for extended amounts of time every day - either for personal pleasure or professional reasons - then you can avoid back pain resulting from neck strain by keeping your head level and bringing the documents up to that level. Keeping your head bent or raised at unnatural angles for extended amounts of time can cause strain. So having a document hanger or holding your materials up instead of setting them on a desk or in your lap can help to prevent

cumulative neck injuries related to these posture no-no's.

105.   Both very active occupations and also jobs in which there is minimal movement can be detrimental to your back. Constantly lifting, pushing and maneuvering in odd ways can really hurt your back and you should always pay attention to your movements. Also, not moving often enough can also cause a lot of back pain if you do not take the proper precautions.

106.   Try not to stand for long periods of time. Doing this can cause a back injury because of all the strain that you are putting your body through. If you have a job that causes you to be on your feet all day, make sure to sit on your breaks, and when you get home you rest for a little.

107.   If you have back pain you should sleep on a firm mattress. If you find that your mattress is not firm enough you can place plywood between the mattress and box spring to stiffen it. The firm surface will provide the support necessary for your back. A soft mattress allows your bones and joints to become misaligned.

108.    If you have back pain and have the money for it, consider paying for a visit to the chiropractor. Chiropractors are trained in many different ways to help minimize pain in your body and many specialize in back pain. If it works out financially, a trip to the chiropractor might just cure what ails your back.

109.    One of the actions you can do to help relieve back pain is to strengthen your core. Do sit-ups and any other form of exercise that will strengthen your abdominal core, which in turn will help ease your back pain. Make sure you do each exercise correctly, though. You certainly do not want to cause yourself more pain.

110.    Back pain can most often be the result of being overweight. Start off walking; adding time and mileage to your treks. When you can actually breathe while walking, start a strength and flexibility program. To make sure you keep on task, drag a friend along with you, or if you don't have a friend available, pop in a DVD in your living room.

111.    Sometimes, no matter what precautions you take, you can end up with that annoying back pain. What do you do? You should get off your

feet and lay flat on your back. Also, drink plenty of fluids, preferably water. The water helps release toxins that hinder the pain in your muscles.

112.    Many women suffer from back pain during pregnancy. A growing baby changes your center of gravity and causes you to lean back to counteract this, causing pain in the lower back. The best remedy for this is good posture. Sit straight and keep your shoulders back. Sit in a comfortable chair and relax. Baby your back while you wait for baby!

113.    There can be many causes for back pain and you will want to be sure to identify what is causing the pain before you try to do anything to resolve it. Try changing up some minor things in your life to see if these have any effect on your pain.

114.    One of the leading causes of back pain actually seems like one of the most harmless jobs. This is having a desk job and sitting in front of a computer all day. Your posture is probably very bad at this job and you do not get much movement, leading to back pain.

115.    A relatively newer type of treatment for back problems, low level laser therapy (3LT) may be a great way to help you get rid of back pain. These cold lasers are noninvasive and can help assist the problems at a cellular level. As little as one treatment can relieve the symptoms of back pain.

116.    To get instant, lasting pain relief for serious back injuries, you need to get a prescription from a doctor. Unfortunately, over-the-counter pain relief is not designed to treat chronic back pain caused by serious injuries like ruptured discs. If you cannot get to your chiropractor right away, then ask your regular doctor about getting a prescription for oxycodone or morphine.

117.    Exercise regularly to increase your core's strength. Make sure to focus on your abs and back muscles. Incorporate plenty of strength and flexibility exercises into your exercise regimen to help you keep your core strong and flexible, which reduces the risk for back pain to develop in the future.

118.    Believe it or not, sleep is actually an essential part of healing from back injuries. Your body does most of its repair work at night when you are relaxed and sleeping and can dedicate all of your energy to healing. If you are experiencing

chronic back pain, then good sleep is as important as good medicine.

119.    Muscle spasms must be calmed to help with back pain. Lying down and applying heat to the muscles is the fastest way to ease your pain. It is also a good idea to reduce how much sodium you eat and drink and instead drink a ton of water. Too much salt and not enough liquids can cause dehydration, which can trigger muscle spasm or make them worse.

120.    Although many people believe otherwise, people who have back pain must exercise frequently. Some people are inclined to believe that exercising will increase back pain, but it really can be quite helpful. When the muscles in the back get stretched out, it can help soothe the pain for a lot of people.

121.    Laying comfortably might not be the best thing for your back. Slouching can feel rather relaxing, but it is important not to do this because it works your muscles harder than it does when you do not slouch.

122.    Be careful about the way you sleep. Sleeping flat on your back not only prevents you from straining it during the night, but also allows you

to position a heating pad under you. Don't ever sleep on your stomach.

123.   One of the best ways to ease your back pain is to flip. Flip your mattress. The springs and inner build up of your mattress can settle over time. Turn your mattress clockwise. Next time, flip it completely over. By doing this it will help your mattress wear evenly which will ease your pain.

124.   Undoubtedly, one of the best possible methods to relieve back pain is to exercise regularly. You do not have to become a cardio enthusiast or a quasi weight-lifter, but exercising every day will work wonders in relieving back pain associated with cramping muscles. The physical activity can really help to get rid of the pain.

125.   If you want to get rid of a large portion of back pain, stop situations where spasms are triggered. Use proper posture, practice safe methods for lifting heavy items, don't overuse your muscles and drink an adequate amount of water to avoid back pain caused by muscle spasms. Applying heat or massaging the area will relax muscles and increase blood flow to stop a back spasm.

126.   One of the leading causes of back pain actually seems like one of the most harmless jobs. This is having a desk job and sitting in front of a computer all day. Your posture is probably very bad at this job and you do not get much movement, leading to back pain.

127.   Back pain can be caused by so many things that it is often very difficult to identify what is causing it. Be sure to talk to a doctor and have him walk you through your routine, including sleeping positions. Hopefully he will be able to find some potential causes.

128.   One of the most common and unexpected causes of bad back pain is your sleeping position. Many people are not aware of exactly how they sleep and this can easily cause you to twist your back into bad positions. Be sure to discuss this possibility with your doctor or physician.

129.   You should know that the proper sleep can help you to get rid of back pain, but more important is the actually position in which you're sleeping. Make sure that you're not tossing and turning and make sure that your body is aligned properly while you're sleeping. A great pillow and

comfortable mattress go a long way to helping you keep back pain at bay.

130.    Before you begin to exercise or do any other type of physical activity, you should always warm up to prevent muscle pulls and cramping. Even if you're only going for a light jog or a walk around the block, a muscle cramp in your lower back can cause excruciating pain that will not soon subside.

131.    Willow bark and Devil's claw are two holistic medications that are taken orally to ease back pain. There is a long list of different products you could buy, and the stores all sell different products. Chiropractic care, acupuncture and massages are alternative remedies for relieving back pain.

132.    If your belly protrudes, especially during pregnancy, stomach-sleeping is out. Likewise, back-sleeping is also a bad idea because of the strain it places on your back. Positioning yourself on either side solves this problem by distributing your weight fairly evenly.

133.    Put heat on any back spasms. Make a warm compress or get a heating pad and just relax. It can soothe the muscles and relax you. Stress can

be a large part of back pain, so just laying down and trying to relax can end up doing wonders for you.

134.    If you're suffering from back pain, be sure to stretch regularly. Stretching can prevent back pain from occurring at all. It can also ease existing back pain. If your back pain is intense, you will probably want to meet with your doctor before adding too much strenuous activity to your daily routine. Otherwise, stretching is usually a great idea.

135.    Make sure you're maintaining a proper weight. If you're overweight, particularly if that weight is in your upper body, you'll be putting a lot more pressure on your back and spine. By keeping an optimum weight, you'll make sure you're not putting too much stress on your back and spine.

136.    It is important to know and understand whether your back pain is chronic or acute. Chronic back pain lasts for more than three months and is a continuous back pain usually from the result of an injury or illness. Acute back pain can also come from an injury and for other reasons and usually comes on fast and lasts for only a short period of time.

137.  Even being 10 pounds overweight causes problems, so take the initiative to lose those pounds. Carrying additional weight, especially in your abdominal area, can shift your body's center of gravity. This weight can strain your lower back, and even lead to chronic back pain.

138.  Depending on the situation, back pain can be such a chronic issue that money can also be a problem. Even with the best of insurance, back problems can really take its toll. Therefore, it is best while attempting costly avenues to also make sure that you are doing everything you can that is less costly and also still effective.

139.  If you are deficient in vitamin B-12, you may be at risk for back pain. Studies show that this vitamin can alleviate low back pain. People who receive vitamin B-12 injections, show a statistically significant reduction in pain and disability. Meat and dairy products are some other good ways to get vitamin B-12.

140.  Many women suffer from back pain during pregnancy. A growing baby changes your center of gravity and causes you to lean back to counteract this, causing pain in the lower back. The best remedy for this is good posture. Sit

straight and keep your shoulders back. Sit in a comfortable chair and relax. Baby your back while you wait for baby!

141.    Back pain can be caused by a whole myriad of issues, but one of the most common and easiest things to fix is a poor diet. If you suffer from certain types of back aches, it may be because you have a bad diet or one that is very high in sodium.

142.    For a lighter amount of back pain one good option that you have is to get a massage. This can be a great way to relax and remove the symptoms of the back pain, but remember that it will do nothing to help with the causes of why you have this pain.

143.    Back pain can be caused by so many things that it is often very difficult to identify what is causing it. Be sure to talk to a doctor and have him walk you through your routine, including sleeping positions. Hopefully he will be able to find some potential causes.

144.    If you're one of the many millions of people suffering from back pain, a great and quick remedy you can try is to do squats. Stand straight up with your feet about shoulder's width apart,

and then squat straight down. This will stretch your muscles out and should help to relieve any pain you're feeling.

145.    A great tip you can use to prevent back pain before it starts is to take it easy on the alcoholic beverages. Alcohol will cause you to become dehydrated. This is what causes the hangover. When you become dehydrated, your muscles can become tense, cramp and spasm and ultimately cause pain.

146.    If you can, try to avoid those specialty products and molded pillows and the like to assist in relieving back pain. These cause your body to conform to a certain position, and once you're no longer in this position, the pain can return. Simply put, it's just a waste of money. You can relieve back pain on your own.

147.    Some back pain is tolerable and is not the sign of anything actually wrong with your body, so a great remedy to alleviate it is to simply take your mind off of it. Soak in a warm tub or listen to some music with mild back pain until it passes. Dwelling on it may make it worse.

148.    It's always great to find some kind of lumbar support if you have back pain, so roll up a towel

to put behind your back when you sit down. Having this type of support for your back will help to alleviate and maybe even help to eliminate lower back pain in most people.

149.   Being overweight can lead to back problems. Having to carry around extra weight puts a lot of strain on the back. If you do need to lose a couple of pounds to help your back feel better, set small goals for yourself so that you can achieve success often.

150.   To determine your back pain's severity and to avoid worsening the injury, try resting for a couple days after you experience pain. If the pain decreases, most likely the injury was minor. Now if the pain is still there or it has increased, then it would be highly advisable that you seek a professional chiropractor or doctor to figure out the source of this pain. Resting for more than 48 hours usually won't do any good, and it may even make the problem worse due to back muscle atrophy.

151.   To aid your body in healing from painful back injuries, invest in a firm mattress. Many people mistakenly believe that a soft mattress will be more comforting to their injured back. In truth, a soft mattress will not help you to

maintain your posture through the night while a firm mattress gives your back the support it needs to repair itself.

152.   To help prevent back pain, have adequate back support when lounging. Furniture isn't always designed with this in mind, so remember to use good posture and back support when sitting and reclining. For example, give your lower back a little support by placing a rolled up towel in the small of your back.

153.   Try not to stand for long periods of time. Doing this can cause a back injury because of all the strain that you are putting your body through. If you have a job that causes you to be on your feet all day, make sure to sit on your breaks, and when you get home you rest for a little.

154.   Eating a healthy diet not only helps keep your weight at a good level, but also a balanced healthy diet with plenty of Vitamin D keeps your bones strong which means your back stays strong. A balanced diet is important for every aspect of health, so not surprisingly, it is no different with your back health.

155.   For severe back pain caused by trauma or degeneration, surgery may be required. Surgery should be considered as a last resort, only when all other options have failed. Surgery could be the only option for certain conditions and injuries that may cause back pain.

156.   If you have back pain you should sleep on a firm mattress. If you find that your mattress is not firm enough you can place plywood between the mattress and box spring to stiffen it. The firm surface will provide the support necessary for your back. A soft mattress allows your bones and joints to become misaligned.

157.   In order to prevent back strains, do not lift anything too heavy. Many times, chronic back pain is caused by someone picking up objects that are too heavy which strains their back. You can avoid this pain by only lifting objects that you know your body, and more specifically, your back, can handle.

158.   Chiropractors are able to try and heal back pain and prevent further back pain by realigning a person's spinal column. They are back specialists and therefore very confident in their abilities to help improve one's back and provide the necessary healing process. Chiropractors can

be very efficient in helping you get rid of your back pain.

159.    Believe it or not, drinking coffee can help to ease chronic back pain. New medical studies showed caffeine in coffee blocks the chemical adenosine. Adenosine tightens your back muscles. By drinking coffee, you are preventing that from happening and helping your muscles stay flexible.

160.    One of the best back pain remedies you can find is a simple hot shower. By standing in the shower and allowing hot water to flow over your back, your muscles will begin to relax. Even for something like a slipped disc, a hot shower will work wonders. Just be careful not to slip and cause more damage.

161.    What you're sleeping on might be responsible for the back pain you're dealing with, so always thoroughly check your mattress to see if you should make a change. Maybe you can get by with a memory foam mattress pad, or maybe you will have to replace the entire mattress. Either way, it's important to take care of the issue to take care of your back.

162.   Back pain sufferers sometimes have a lot of trouble getting around, but you should still try to perform activities like swimming in order to relieve the pain. Swimming is really a full-body workout, and it definitely helps to stretch and loosen the muscles in the back. Plus the water is soothing for your back.

163.   Prevent any situations which can cause your back to have fits, and you will get rid of a major cause of your back pain. Use proper posture, practice safe methods for lifting heavy items, don't overuse your muscles and drink an adequate amount of water to avoid back pain caused by muscle spasms. If you do develop a back spasm, apply heat to the area and rest your back to avoid developing more debilitating pain.

164.   Maintaining good posture is something that you should always strive for, but it is especially important in this position. Straighten your back, keep your feet flat with one slightly in front of the other foot, and have your elbows down at your side. Maintaining the proper position of your neck is important, too. Never look down or stretch your neck in order to properly view your computer screen. If you must do this, try to find a new position for the screen.

165.    Use ice to help alleviate back pain, as it can reduce swelling and inflammation from injuries that cause back pain. Apply the ice to the affected area two or three times per day for 10 to 20 minutes, and this may help you feel better. An ice pack or a bag of frozen vegetables can be used for this purpose.

166.    Don't stress out about a new back pain. Lower back pain is very common, especially among middle-aged Americans. It is unlikely to be an indicator of a more serious disease or condition, and it will likely clear up over time even if it is not treated by a medical professional.

167.    Unnecessary back pain can be caused by poor posture. If sitting or standing, maintain good posture. Assuming that back pain is only the result of injury from physical activity is just not true. Sitting with poor posture for a long time, as people often do when working at a computer, can damage the muscles of the back.

168.    Pain in the lower back is the most common type of back pain and is second on the list of reasons why people see a doctor. Many times there are things that you could be doing differently in your everyday life that will help reduce back pain. Make sure that you are always

taking the necessary precautions to protect your back. It your lower back pain is inevitable, you can still try to prevent it.

169.    Do not wear a shoe with a heel over one inch. If heels higher than this are worn, the wearer's center of gravity shifts. This causes back strain and pain. It can become chronic pain if high heels are worn often. If they must be worn, limiting the amount of time spent in them will help decrease the chance of pain and injury.

170.    Quitting smoking can help to ease back pain. People who smoke, especially heavy smokers, do not have as much blood flow to the spine as those who don't smoke. Without a sufficient amount of blood flow to the spine, your back will hurt.

171.    Heat has also been found to be an effective way to relieve back problems, especially lower back pain. Heat therapy, such as heating pads, wraps or baths are inespensive and easy to do. It's best to alternate back and forth between ice and heat therapy to get the best results.

172.    When you hurt your back, usually hamstring stretching exercises can prove to be very helpful. If the muscles on the backs of your thighs are

tight, they can usually cause your lower back to experience a lot of unnecessary stress and pain. You should stretch your hamstring muscles at least twice a day for 45 seconds at a time.

173.    One of the absolute best ways to strengthen your back is to keep it flexible. Yoga, Pilates or Tai Chi are some methods that will help you. Two to four times a week, alternated with strength training will put you in tip top shape. Give it some time and soon you will hopefully forget the pain that had you lying on the couch.

174.    One of the best back pain remedies you can find is a simple hot shower. By standing in the shower and allowing hot water to flow over your back, your muscles will begin to relax. Even for something like a slipped disc, a hot shower will work wonders. Just be careful not to slip and cause more damage.

175.    Mind your posture at all times. Your back should always be straight, and both feet should be resting on the floor with one a bit ahead. When typing, keep elbows resting comfortably at your sides. See to it that you're not looking down and that you are not craning your neck when staring at your computer screen.

176.   Some methods are better to try than others when fighting against back pain, and one of the best you can try is to simply elevate your legs. By lying flat on your back and elevating your legs, you are taking a whole heap of tension off of your back muscles. This will allow for the muscles to relax.

177.   Spending such a significant amount of time in your car actually contributes to back pain. Adjust the seat properly, where you can sit comfortably, but not so much that it causes you to develop bad posture or slack off.

178.   People with anxiety issues can become tense, this can lead to muscle strains and spasms and then lead to back pain. Work on various ways to overcome your anxiety with relaxation techniques and as an added bonus you can get rid of back pain.

179.   Sleeping in a good position that works for your body will help to reduce straining of your back at night. Use your comfort to be your guide, and don't try to sleep in a certain position because you heard it was the right thing to do. Everybody is different, and will have different needs.

180.  If you're riding in the car for long periods, try putting a towel in the arch of your back for extra support. Also, make sure to move your seat a little forward or back every once in a while so that your spine has a chance to move and doesn't get stiff.

181.  Look at how you walk. Actually, have your doctor watch you walk. Many times people can develop back pain because of a gait irregularity. This is simple to fix, you will just need to go to physical therapy for a short time until the problem is corrected. Many insurance plans will cover physical therapy, though it's always wise to give them a call first to make sure.

182.  If your back pain gets to be too debilitating, consider seeking professional help. If you have insurance, there is a good chance it might cover a few sessions. Trained physical therapists can give you helpful advice and help you to develop an exercise regimen that will work to strengthen your back.

183.  Use ice to help alleviate back pain, as it can reduce swelling and inflammation from injuries that cause back pain. Apply the ice to the affected area two or three times per day for 10 to 20 minutes, and this may help you feel better. An

ice pack or a bag of frozen vegetables can be used for this purpose.

184.    Maintain proper posture in order to prevent back pain. It is important to stand, sit and walk properly so that your muscles and ligaments do not pull your vertebrae out of alignment and cause pain. Your head, neck and spine should be aligned properly at all times to help prevent any pain.

185.    After you're finished exercising, make sure you stretch. This will help keep your muscles loose and limber and prevent them from tightening up. Having muscles that are overly tight is a very common source of back pain so you want to avoid that. By stretching as a cool down, you'll be able to keep those muscles loose.

186.    If you are having back pain while you working on the computer try this, make sure arms are comfortable. Raising your arms or extending them on a keyboard that is placed too high can cause back strain. Adjust your keyboard to a comfortable level to reduce the strain on your upper back.

187.    Clean out your purse, backpack or briefcase on a regular basis. Depending on the size and

how often you use the item, you may need to clean it out weekly. It is easy to accumulate unnecessary items over time. The less weight you carry, the more healthy your back will be.

188.    No matter what the reason, if you suffer from back pain and you have to bend over, be sure to do so with your knees and not your back. Many people suffer from back strains or pains because they bend over using their back, which puts too much pressure on the spine.

189.    A great way to fight against back pain is to actually fight against your stress levels. Having high levels of stress can easily trigger a back spasm or general back pain. Even if it's psychosomatic, the pain is still real enough, so remember to try to get rid of your stress in order to get rid of back pain.

190.    If you have chronic back pain and cannot figure out how to get rid of it, perhaps a new chair is in order, like a recliner or something softer than what you're sitting on now. A lot of people think that firm support is a must, but that's more to prevent pain. If you need to relieve it, go with something soft.

191.    Your back pain could be a distant memory if
you have access to a vibrating chair. These chairs
are usually equipped different strength levels of
the vibrating system as well as being able to hone
in on certain areas of your back. As a bonus,
your chair might heat up, too!

192.    For people who experience chronic back
pain, your first visit shouldn't be to the store to
purchase a massager but rather to the doctor's
office to see if you have a slipped disc or another
type of injury. Back pain can be the result of a
hundred different things, and many of them can
be serious.

193.    They say that most things are a case of mind
over matter, and this can definitely be true for
back pain. So when you're struck with some
minor pain, a great remedy here is to try some
aromatherapy techniques or other relaxation
techniques to see if you can eliminate the pain.

194.    It is important that you learn to identify the
difference in physical exertion and physical pain
if you want to get rid of back pain. At the onset
of pain, you can begin to do a few stretches to
loosen your muscles. With exertion, you will
know that it's time to take a rest before you
injure yourself.

195.   Taking a long, brisk walk can help you to loosen up your muscles and eliminate the back pain you're dealing with. While walking might not actually cure the pain permanently, the exercise will help soothe the pain by stretching the muscles and keeping them warm. Take the dog around the block or walk to the store and back.

196.   Avoid very hard soled shoes if you are suffering from back pain. Hard soled shoes can cause compression problems with your spinal cord. The result can be painful flare ups in your lower back. Try a comfortable pair of orthopedic shoes, or even a simple pair of running shoes, instead.

197.   When required to sit in the same position for an extended period, be sure to cross your legs frequently. When your legs are crossed, your muscles in your back and hip are used, so these muscles are doing something even when sitting. Alternate crossing your legs so you use all of your muscles.

198.   A good, professional massage therapist can loosen your back muscles and keep the pain from causing you any limitations. The majority

of back pain is a result of simple day-to-day life and stress. A good massage helps your back recover from the daily stresses and is an investment in the long term, helping control your back pain.

199.   Use ice to help alleviate back pain, as it can reduce swelling and inflammation from injuries that cause back pain. Apply the ice to the affected area two or three times per day for 10 to 20 minutes, and this may help you feel better. An ice pack or a bag of frozen vegetables can be used for this purpose.

200.   Use over the counter pain relievers, such as ibuprofen and acetaminophen, to help relieve back pain. Taking oral pain medications can allow you to function somewhat normally when you are suffering from a bout of back pain. Be sure to follow the instructions on the package for best results.

201.   If back injuries are something that you are prone to getting, either through genetics or lifestyle choices, make sure you see the chiropractor on a regular basis, even before the onset of pain. A chiropractor can fix any small issues before they turn into serious injuries.

202.	To aid your body in healing from painful back injuries, invest in a firm mattress. Many people mistakenly believe that a soft mattress will be more comforting to their injured back. In truth, a soft mattress will not help you to maintain your posture through the night while a firm mattress gives your back the support it needs to repair itself.

203.	While breast augmentation is the more common procedure, more and more women are opting for breast reduction. It is necessary more often than you might think, though. Extremely large breasts can strain your back, resulting in back pain. Women that receive breast implants often discover this burden.

204.	Learning to lift properly can save yourself a lot of back pain in the future. Learning to lift from the knees instead of just bending over to lift will greatly reduce the strain on your back. This will keep your back from being over exerted and help you keep your back from developing pain earlier.

205.	When battling the discomfort of back pain, allowing yourself to become stressed about it will not do any good at all. You must learn how to properly relax so you don't increase the risk of developing muscle spasms. Get enough rest, and you may find heat relaxing to your muscles.

206.   Many times taking an over the counter pain medicine will help ease back pain. You may have to take it for a couple days, and then you will notice the pain is gone. Make sure you read the directions to the pills very carefully, and don't take to much thinking it will work faster.

207.   How many times have you seen a woman carrying a heavy purse on one shoulder? How many times have you seen a student carrying his or her backpack on one shoulder? You should always make heavy loads proportionate, and also make sure to limit the amount of time you have to carry them on a consistent basis.

208.   Be sure that you wear comfortable sneakers or shoes if you suffer from back pain. Walking with heels or other uncomfortable shoes can make you walk improperly and cause back pain to begin or increase. Try to buy sneakers that are fitting and have a rubber sole on the bottom for the best support.

209.   Proper stretching is probably one of the best ways you can work to eliminate frequent back pain. When you stretch, whether you're doing toe

touches, sit-ups or side bends, you are loosening the muscles and relieving some of the tension there. A failure to stretch properly could lead to a pulled muscle or spasms.

210.   For a lighter amount of back pain one good option that you have is to get a massage. This can be a great way to relax and remove the symptoms of the back pain, but remember that it will do nothing to help with the causes of why you have this pain.

211.   It's always great to find some kind of lumbar support if you have back pain, so roll up a towel to put behind your back when you sit down. Having this type of support for your back will help to alleviate and maybe even help to eliminate lower back pain in most people.

212.   You may be tempted to get up and walk around with a hurt back, thinking you can fight through the pain, but it is imperative that you give your injury proper time to heal. A pulled, strained or torn muscle will only hurt twice as much and take twice as long to heal if it's aggravated.

213.   If you're wearing a backpack, make sure that you wear it properly if you want to eliminate

back pain. You should not wear these packs on your shoulders. The straps are for your shoulders. The actual body of the pack should be closer to your lower back so that the weight is spread evenly.

214.	Taking a warm bath can help relive any type of musculoskeletal pain. Warm water tends to be very soothing. Spend about 20 minutes in the tub a day, and if your back is really bad you can do this a couple of times a day (as long as your skin is okay). Adding some aromatherapy oil can also be helpful.

215.	If your job involves standing still for long periods of time, this can be a major cause of back strain. One method of reducing this strain is to have a prop like a box or small footstool to alternately put your foot on. This relaxes some muscles and stretches the back.

216.	Don't ignore the pain. If you know a particular activity is going to exacerbate your pain, then don't do that activity. Ignoring it will not make it go away faster. In fact, pushing through the pain will probably result in further injury, making the pain last even longer.

217.    Practice retaining good posture, even when sitting, in order to prevent needless back pain. A lot of people think that strenuous physical activity is the only cause of back injury. Truthfully, even long periods of improper sitting like the bad postures people often have in front of computers can add up to back injury.

218.    If you sit for long periods of time, keep your feet slightly elevated on a stool or on a stack of books. Doing this will help keep your back aligned correctly and keep pressure from building. Make sure to take breaks, as well and work out those muscles.

219.    Wear comfortable low-heeled shoes. The stress that high-heeled shoes put on your ankles and legs is transmitted up your body all the way to your hips and spine. Comfortable shoes will allow you to stand and walk more naturally, which can greatly reduce your incidence of back pain the next morning.

220.    Do not let your back pain stress you out; this only makes the pain worse. Learning to relax helps to ease the tension in your muscles which will decrease the chances of another injury. Apply a heat source to the affected area of your back, then allow yourself to rest.

221.    To prevent getting back pain, you need to make sure that you exercise on a regular basis. This will help increase and strengthen the muscles in your back. You just need to be careful that you are not lifting weights that are too heavy and that you are not doing anything else that could actually cause an injury.

222.    One area of your life that can be affected by chronic back pain is your sex life. If left covered up, you are not allowing your partner to be understanding of your back pain. Your partner may think another reason is putting a strain on you guys' sex life. Therefore, it is imperative to be open and honest and look for ways for your back pain not to disrupt your sex life.

223.    When you hurt your back, usually hamstring stretching exercises can prove to be very helpful. If the muscles on the backs of your thighs are tight, they can usually cause your lower back to experience a lot of unnecessary stress and pain. You should stretch your hamstring muscles at least twice a day for 45 seconds at a time.

224.    Back pain can be debilitating, both physically as well as emotionally. Yoga has been proved to reduce pain, use of pain medication, and

disability. Yoga develops flexibility and strength, creating balance in the body. When the body is out of balance, pain is the result.

225.    When working at your desk or computer, make sure you sit in the proper posture or purchase an ergonomic chair. Be sure to get up and walk around and loosen your muscles. It is easier to keep them from getting cramped rather than trying to get out the cramps in your back.

226.    Obesity has been shown to be an important factor in chronic back pain. Losing pounds and keeping weight within normal ranges can greatly reduce pain and strain on the back. Regular exercise can also help strengthen back muscles. These are the top recommendations by doctors to obese patients suffering from back pain.

227.    If you want to eliminate back pain, you should try to stay properly hydrated. Drinking plenty of water is great for your overall health, but it is especially good for your muscle health. Muscles are essentially water and protein, and once you start to become dehydrated. Your muscles can easily spasm.

228.    In some cases, back pain sufferers find that acupuncture is a good treatment for their

ailment. The jury is still out on acupuncture, and it might be a little too pricy depending on how available it is in your area, but thousands of back pain sufferers swear by the results of the needles.

229.    Before you begin to exercise or do any other type of physical activity, you should always warm up to prevent muscle pulls and cramping. Even if you're only going for a light jog or a walk around the block, a muscle cramp in your lower back can cause excruciating pain that will not soon subside.

230.    Always avoid any back surgery unless it is absolutely necessary. Sometimes a slipped disc can be surgically repaired, but there may be other ways to treat it. Some will opt for the surgery because they believe it's a quicker fix for back pain, but anything can go wrong under the knife.

231.    One common cause of back pain that many people don't consider is the weight of the arms tiring the upper back and shoulders. If you have a job that requires you to sit for long periods, make sure to have a chair with arm rests, and use them frequently.

232.    Think a 135 degree angle instead of 90 degree angle while sitting. Many people think the

proper angle for sitting is 90 degrees, but researchers have found that the most optimum angle for sitting is actually 135 degrees. Sitting at 135 degrees puts much less strain on your back, which in affect will lower your back pain.

233.    Use over the counter pain relievers, such as ibuprofen and acetaminophen, to help relieve back pain. Taking oral pain medications can allow you to function somewhat normally when you are suffering from a bout of back pain. Be sure to follow the instructions on the package for best results.

234.    If you suffer from problems with back pain, heat and ice your back. In the first two to three days of back pain, you want to put ice on it to reduce the inflammation. Aafter the first three days of icing your back you want to apply heat to loosen and relax your muscles.

235.    Most people complain of lower back pain than upper back pain. It may be that your daily routine is contributing to your back pain, so a few simple changes can provide some relief. Lower back pain might seem like it is something that is bound to happen to you, so you should take steps to prevent it!

236.    Both very active occupations and also jobs in which there is minimal movement can be detrimental to your back. Constantly lifting, pushing and maneuvering in odd ways can really hurt your back and you should always pay attention to your movements. Also, not moving often enough can also cause a lot of back pain if you do not take the proper precautions.

237.    While anesthetic and steroid shots are common for back pain, this is not effective for everyone. In addition, prolonged episodes of this can actually sometimes cause more back pain to the person. However, these methods are popular and necessary for treatment of back pain in some scenarios. Again, it is your physician that will determine the treatment.

238.    If you have back pain you should sleep on a firm mattress. If you find that your mattress is not firm enough you can place plywood between the mattress and box spring to stiffen it. The firm surface will provide the support necessary for your back. A soft mattress allows your bones and joints to become misaligned.

239.    Going to a chiropractor can be a generally scary experience if you are not familiar. However, it is also a very eye opening and

relieving experience as well. However, you should not go to just any chiropractor. Go to a well-respected one, and make sure that who touches your back is highly qualified and not messing it up further.

240.    It may seem odd, but you can find relief from your back pain by having a cup of coffee. Studies are pointing to the caffeine found in coffee blocking a chemical named adenosine. Adenosine can cause back stiffness, so coffee drinking may help you stretch your back muscles, resulting in less pain.

241.    Be mindful of the position you sleep in. While a prone sleeping position may not be your favorite option, it can help you to avoid back pain. For added relief, you may place a heating pad under your body. Make sure that you do not sleep on your stomach.

242.    Use ice! If you have back pain from a legitimate injury "" and not just a muscle cramp or basic tension - use an ice pack to relieve the pain! Ice is a natural pain reliever for many ailments, and the cold will help to reduce any swelling associated with any injuries you may be suffering!

243.   Back pain can be caused by so many things that it is often very difficult to identify what is causing it. Be sure to talk to a doctor and have him walk you through your routine, including sleeping positions. Hopefully he will be able to find some potential causes.

244.   In order to help reduce your back pain, try to eat a diet higher in potassium. Food items like bananas are great for your muscles. Potassium is a vital mineral that your body needs, and athletes have used potassium to keep from cramping for hundreds of years. It can certainly help to alleviate back pain.

245.   Doing the simple things can help you alleviate back pain, like simply taking your time when you stand up or get out of bed. Sudden movements and jerking motions can jar the muscles and even cause discs to slip and slide around. Be cognizant of your movements and take a little time when getting up.

246.   A solid 20% of all back pain-related tips you read suggest you check your mattress, but you should also check what's under your mattress. Sometimes your mattress isn't enough to support your back. You need a solid box spring under

there. Don't go with only the support of the mattress top.

247.    When you are lifting heavy objects, always lift at the knee. Bend your knees every time you reach down. If you bend at your waist, your chances of hurting your back are much higher. If you need to lift heavy objects often, you should wear a back brace to protect your back even further.

248.    Many people develop back problems by having a poorly constructed computer setup. Working at a computer for long periods of time with back pain requires that you take preventive measures, such as placing the screen in a direct frontal position and having the monitor at the level of your eyes.

249.    Do some yoga. Yoga is a great way to not only relax and de-stress, but to deal with back pain as well. Yoga is made up of different positions that ease back pain by gently stretching muscles. Getting into a good yoga practices is a consistent way to tackle back pain.

250.    To help prevent or alleviate back pain, try walking each day. Research has indicated that walking helps relieve back pain, whereas doing

specific exercises meant to alleviate back pain may actually make the pain worse. Although your back may hurt, it is important to walk briskly for three hours per week to obtain relief.

251.   The right workout routine can help you rehab and reduce back injuries and their resulting pain. For instance, practicing yoga regularly will strengthen your back and make it more flexible. On the other hand, some exercises focus on the core, helping take the burden off the back when lifting or other such activities.

252.   If you're suffering from back pain, be sure to stretch regularly. Stretching can prevent back pain from occurring at all. It can also ease existing back pain. If your back pain is intense, you will probably want to meet with your doctor before adding too much strenuous activity to your daily routine. Otherwise, stretching is usually a great idea.

253.   Even with severe back pain, if you stress a lot over it, you just make yourself feel worse. Instead, discover ways to relax so there is less chance you will experience spasms in your back muscles. Get enough rest, and you may find heat relaxing to your muscles.

254.   It is important to know and understand whether your back pain is chronic or acute. Chronic back pain lasts for more than three months and is a continuous back pain usually from the result of an injury or illness. Acute back pain can also come from an injury and for other reasons and usually comes on fast and lasts for only a short period of time.

255.   Having back pain? Get a massage. Getting a back massage will ease the sore tensed muscles in your back, and help to relieve the stress of back pain. Having a 30 minute massage either by a professional or a family member can produce long lasting relief from sore back muscles.

256.   It is important to learn how to lift safely in order to avoid back pain and injury. When you lift safely, you use the large muscles in your legs to spare your back. Bend at the knees, suck your stomach in and keep the item close to your body as you lift.

257.   If you are more than ten pounds over your ideal weight then you need to go on a diet to reduce your weight. Extra weight, particularly in the abdominal area, shifts your center of gravity. That puts a strain on your lower back, and as time passes can result in chronic lower back pain.

258.    In order to heal your back, you must remove yourself from the source of pain. Once removed, then find yourself a place to rest. Whether it be a comfortable chair, recliner or even a place to lay down. Find a position that offers you the most support to relieve your back tension.

259.    Back pain can be debilitating, both physically as well as emotionally. Yoga has been proved to reduce pain, use of pain medication, and disability. Yoga develops flexibility and strength, creating balance in the body. When the body is out of balance, pain is the result.

260.    A great way to fight against back pain is to actually fight against your stress levels. Having high levels of stress can easily trigger a back spasm or general back pain. Even if it's psychosomatic, the pain is still real enough, so remember to try to get rid of your stress in order to get rid of back pain.

261.    Proper stretching is probably one of the best ways you can work to eliminate frequent back pain. When you stretch, whether you're doing toe touches, sit-ups or side bends, you are loosening the muscles and relieving some of the tension

there. A failure to stretch properly could lead to a pulled muscle or spasms.

262.    If your back pain does not improve or continues to get worse, you may want to look into a chiropractor. At your initial visit the chiropractor will order x-rays so that he can develop a treatment plan for your condition. If you follow your doctor's suggestions your back pain should decrease over time.

263.    If you are pregnant and suffering from back pain, consider a maternity belt to alleviate some of the discomfort. The growing belly can really make standing straight difficult, but a maternity belt supports the stomach, thereby reducing strain on the back. Comfortable, low-heeled shoes are equally important for good posture.

264.    Sleep in the proper position to prevent back pain and avoid aggravating existing back pain. If you sleep on your side, place a pillow between your knees. If you sleep on your back, try placing the pillow under your knees. A firm mattress will also help to alleviate pain.

265.    Not all back pain is from your muscles or from slipped discs, so be sure that you're not dealing with nerve pain called sciatica. This pain

may not be able to be treated like normal back pain. Make sure you understand the type of back pain you're dealing with if simple remedies don't work.

266.    Work on toning your abdominal muscles to avoid future back pain. Having a strong core will enable you to have good posture and also help prevent your back from getting injured often. Just make sure when you are working your abs, if you start to feel back pain, take a break.

267.    To help prevent or alleviate back pain, try walking each day. Research has indicated that walking helps relieve back pain, whereas doing specific exercises meant to alleviate back pain may actually make the pain worse. Although your back may hurt, it is important to walk briskly for three hours per week to obtain relief.

268.    Maintain proper posture in order to prevent back pain. It is important to stand, sit and walk properly so that your muscles and ligaments do not pull your vertebrae out of alignment and cause pain. Your head, neck and spine should be aligned properly at all times to help prevent any pain.

269.   Avoid repeated stress on the same muscles, no matter what position or stance you are taking. Avoid doing the same repetitive motion over and over again. Shift your weight from foot to foot, and make sure you walk around frequently.

270.   To aid your body in healing from painful back injuries, invest in a firm mattress. Many people mistakenly believe that a soft mattress will be more comforting to their injured back. In truth, a soft mattress will not help you to maintain your posture through the night while a firm mattress gives your back the support it needs to repair itself.

271.   To help reduce swelling and alleviate back pain resulting from muscle strain, try compressing the back muscles. To compress the injured muscles, consider using an elastic bandage or even a back support. The act of compressing the muscles helps decrease the inflammation in the muscles. This, in turn, leads to an easing in back pain.

272.   You may need to lose some weight if you're carrying any extra. Extra weight will shift your body's center of gravity and put stress on your muscles and tendons. This puts more strain on

the lower back which can result in chronic lower back pain.

273.    Your doctor may recommend surgery on your back as a way to help ease your disorder or back pain. Surgery should only be used as a last resort if all other avenues have been exhausted. For certain types of back pain and injuries, surgery is the most effective method.

274.    Clean out your purse, backpack or briefcase on a regular basis. Depending on the size and how often you use the item, you may need to clean it out weekly. It is easy to accumulate unnecessary items over time. The less weight you carry, the more healthy your back will be.

275.    It is important that you do not sleep in the same position each night if you suffer from back pain. By sleeping in the same position all night, you are allowing your spine to stiffen up which can cause back pain. Be sure that you replace your mattress and pillow regularly.

276.    When you hurt your back, usually hamstring stretching exercises can prove to be very helpful. If the muscles on the backs of your thighs are tight, they can usually cause your lower back to experience a lot of unnecessary stress and pain.

You should stretch your hamstring muscles at least twice a day for 45 seconds at a time.

277.   Just like with any other type of illness, regular checkups with your doctor can go a long way in preventing back pain and various back problems. Your doctor is trained to keep an eye out for such complications and symptoms, and he or she can do a lot of things for you.

278.   An acupuncture session can be a great way to temporarily relieve back pain. Just remember that acupuncture is not a long-term solution, but it does provide great temporary relief. Don't be afraid of the long needles they stick in your body, because by the end of the session you will be begging for more.

279.   If you are trying to fight off back pain, try reducing the amount of caffeine you use, or eliminate it altogether. Caffeine has a hand in spasms and you may have inflammation in your muscles. Cutting back on sodas, tea and coffee will eliminate most caffeine from your diet.

280.   Your back pain could be a distant memory if you have access to a vibrating chair. These chairs are usually equipped different strength levels of the vibrating system as well as being able to hone

in on certain areas of your back. As a bonus, your chair might heat up, too!

281.	You should know that the proper sleep can help you to get rid of back pain, but more important is the actually position in which you're sleeping. Make sure that you're not tossing and turning and make sure that your body is aligned properly while you're sleeping. A great pillow and comfortable mattress go a long way to helping you keep back pain at bay.

282.	Relaxing your back isn't good enough if you want to get rid of back pain; you need to relax your entire body. Because your back muscles are so large and connected to every other muscle group, tension in your calf muscles or shoulders can cause the back pain to persist and even to intensify.

283.	If your job involves a lot of sitting at a desk, make sure you have a good, ergonomic chair. While this can be expensive in the short term, have a damaged back can cause a lot of pain and be very expensive to fix. Save the trouble and splurge on a nice chair.

284.	If you have to stand for a long period of time, be sure to change positions frequently in order to avoid back pain. Changing positions will help to allocate the pressure to different areas of your body. If possible, stand on a carpet or rubber mat to further lessen the impact to your body.

285.   Chiropractic adjustments can help alleviate back pain. Chiropractors manipulate the spine using various techniques to help align the spine, thereby relieving back pain. Some chiropractors utilize tools, such as impact guns and electrical stimulation, while others rely solely on physical manipulation. Many people find that this type of approach relieves their back pain.

286.   To get instant, lasting pain relief for serious back injuries, you need to get a prescription from a doctor. Unfortunately, over-the-counter pain relief is not designed to treat chronic back pain caused by serious injuries like ruptured discs. If you cannot get to your chiropractor right away, then ask your regular doctor about getting a prescription for oxycodone or morphine.

287.   Consider switching your most commonly used chair into an ergonomic chair. There are several ergonomically designed chairs these days that are made just for those that are sitting at a desk or sitting up all day. These chairs promote

better positioning within the chair, thus offering a greater amount of comfort and less stress on your back.

288.    After you're finished exercising, make sure you stretch. This will help keep your muscles loose and limber and prevent them from tightening up. Having muscles that are overly tight is a very common source of back pain so you want to avoid that. By stretching as a cool down, you'll be able to keep those muscles loose.

289.    Sometimes we are in too much of a hurry or simply too lazy to lift properly. People attempt to do this all of the time because the want to save time. Always place yourself close to the object that you are trying to move, and do not rush the process.

290.    Wear comfortable low-heeled shoes. The stress that high-heeled shoes put on your ankles and legs is transmitted up your body all the way to your hips and spine. Comfortable shoes will allow you to stand and walk more naturally, which can greatly reduce your incidence of back pain the next morning.

291.    To help reduce swelling and alleviate back pain resulting from muscle strain, try

compressing the back muscles. To compress the injured muscles, consider using an elastic bandage or even a back support. The act of compressing the muscles helps decrease the inflammation in the muscles. This, in turn, leads to an easing in back pain.

292.    Back pains try replacing your shoes. If your shoes are worn out, too big or too small, have no padding or arch support that could be your problem. Footwear affects your spinal placement causing you to have back pain. Replacing your old footwear could save you from having back pain.

293.    Maintain proper posture at all times to alleviate back pain. Many adults have pain from being hunched over and not even realizing it. When you are sitting or standing, make sure that your back is extremely straight. It might feel uncomfortable at first. Although your body will get used to it, and your back will thank you later.

294.    Many times when people have back pain, it is in their lower back. This is also the 2nd most popular reason that many people have to visit the doctor. There are many things that could be done differently to help prevent pain in the lower

back. Since lower back pain is common, you should do all you can to avoid it.

295.    If you can, try avoiding tight jeans or pants, if you suffer from chronic back pain. Tight jeans or pants that effect how you sit down, stand, or even walk, are bad for your posture and can cause new pain in the back or worsen pain that you may already have.

296.    An acupuncture session can be a great way to temporarily relieve back pain. Just remember that acupuncture is not a long-term solution, but it does provide great temporary relief. Don't be afraid of the long needles they stick in your body, because by the end of the session you will be begging for more.

297.    If you want to eliminate back pain, you should try to stay properly hydrated. Drinking plenty of water is great for your overall health, but it is especially good for your muscle health. Muscles are essentially water and protein, and once you start to become dehydrated. Your muscles can easily spasm.

298.    To address back pain, take up yoga. Even if you are in poor physical condition, you can begin with some simple, easy positions that will help

stretch your back muscles and loosen tension. By strengthening and lengthening the muscles of the back and releasing tension in the spine, you will eliminate your back pain.

299.   If you want to avoid any potential back injury or just simply wish to alleviate your current back pain, it is important that you never attempt to bend over from a standing position. Always bend your knees and work to lower your entire body. Allowing your back and its muscles to bear the brunt can cause pain.

300.   Even though many people bend at the hips when lifting heavy items, it is best to use your knees to bend instead. You could seriously injure your back by picking up a heavy item the wrong way. Using your knees and bringing the item close against your body while lifting will use your core muscles and avoid a back strain.

301.   Apply an ice pack to the painful area. Despite its simplicity, an ice pack is one of the most effective methods for reducing back pain. Applying ice or a cold pack to the painful area reduces swelling and blood flow, which also reduces the pain. It can also help relieve stiffness.

302.    Before you can treat your back pain, it is important that you visit your doctor to find out what is causing it. The kind of treatment that will provided for you back mostly depends on what the cause of your back pain is. For instance, if it is arthritis, you may have to see a chiropractor.

303.    Heat has also been found to be an effective way to relieve back problems, especially lower back pain. Heat therapy, such as heating pads, wraps or baths are inespensive and easy to do. It's best to alternate back and forth between ice and heat therapy to get the best results.

304.    If you suffer from back pain, remember to stay aware of your posture when sitting down. This is especially important for those who sit in an office chair all day because slumping over your desk can do a number on your spine. Remember to have the soles of your feet flat on the ground and your back as straight and upright as possible.

305.    A lot of back pain sufferers, find that lying on their stomachs can help to relieve the pain. Most lower back pain comes from strain and stress, and lying on the back can actually intensify this due to the muscle tension. Lying on

your stomach, however, can relax these muscles and relieve the pain.

306.    Eliminate back pain by avoiding anything that may cause your back to spasm. Common back spasm triggers are caffeine, dehydration, stress, anxiety, poor sleep and low sodium levels. When you feel a spasm in you back, it is important to treat it with rest and heat compresses to reduce the pain and prevent further damage.

307.    There can be many causes for back pain and you will want to be sure to identify what is causing the pain before you try to do anything to resolve it. Try changing up some minor things in your life to see if these have any effect on your pain.

308.    Back pain can be caused by a whole myriad of issues, but one of the most common and easiest things to fix is a poor diet. If you suffer from certain types of back aches, it may be because you have a bad diet or one that is very high in sodium.

309.    Keep your posture in mind at all times. Your back should be straight, your feet flat on the floor, with one in front of the other and as you

type, keep your elbows by your sides. Make sure your computer screen is level with your eyes so you don't have to move your neck unnaturally to see it.

310.    If you often wake up with back pain after sleeping, you may need to consider getting a new mattress. A mattress that is too soft or old offers little back support and can be the cause of stiffness. Having your back in a bad position for eight hours every night can easily cause a lot of pain.

311.    A solid 20% of all back pain-related tips you read suggest you check your mattress, but you should also check what's under your mattress. Sometimes your mattress isn't enough to support your back. You need a solid box spring under there. Don't go with only the support of the mattress top.

312.    You can reduce the frequency of back pain when you wear shoes that offer the right fit and support. Ill-fitting shoes that make walking difficult can throw your body out of alignment, resulting in bad posture and discomfort. If you need to wear those kinds of shoes for whatever reason, get insoles and don't wear them for long periods.

313.   Find ways to make your daily work activities more active! Invest in a telephone headset so you can walk around your office during a conference call. Walk to someone's office instead of picking up the phone. These habit changes will get you out of your chair and relieve a lot of back pain in the process.

314.   To get instant, lasting pain relief for serious back injuries, you need to get a prescription from a doctor. Unfortunately, over-the-counter pain relief is not designed to treat chronic back pain caused by serious injuries like ruptured discs. If you cannot get to your chiropractor right away, then ask your regular doctor about getting a prescription for oxycodone or morphine.

315.   There are exercises you can do that will reduce the likelihood of you suffering a back injury. Yoga, and other exercises that promote flexibility, can prevent you from straining a muscle. Also, strength based routines can target your core and are great for people who do a lot of lifting and use their back muscles a lot.

316.   In order to help prevent back pain from occurring, make sure you use chairs properly. For example, many office chairs have controls

for adjusting the height and position of the seat back part of the chair. Utilize these controls to ensure you are getting the most comfortable, back-friendly position possible when using these chairs.

317.   You should be diligent about lifting things correctly, even when you are lifting or nursing your children. Many parents injure their backs when rough housing with their children. Likewise, many new mothers strain their backs while nursing. Pain from these injuries is easily avoided by lifting your children from your knees and by holding them closer to your body.

318.   Some people have to work and stand for long hours at a time. If you must do this, then make sure you try and stand tall and straight. Try and allow your legs to rest too from time to time if possible, perhaps on a stool or bench if you are allowed to do that.

319.   Aging brings about increased risk and inevitability of back pain. Therefore, since age is unavoidable, it should be clear that you should take every other precaution that you can in order to maintain back health and keep the back pain away. While age will always be at play, so will all

the other things that you are doing to help yourself.

320.    Eating a healthy diet not only helps keep your weight at a good level, but also a balanced healthy diet with plenty of Vitamin D keeps your bones strong which means your back stays strong. A balanced diet is important for every aspect of health, so not surprisingly, it is no different with your back health.

321.    If you suffer from back pain and you smoke, you need to quit as soon as possible. One of the nasty side effects of smoking is the intake of nicotine. Nicotine reduces blood flow throughout your body, including to your spine, and that increases your risk of back pain.

322.    Buy a bag, purse or backpack with a long strap that can be worn on the opposite shoulder as the item. This allows the weight of the bag to be distributed more evenly across both sides of your body. It also helps keep the shoulders aligned, which helps keep your back from injury.

323.    If you can, try avoiding tight jeans or pants, if you suffer from chronic back pain. Tight jeans or pants that effect how you sit down, stand, or even walk, are bad for your posture and can

cause new pain in the back or worsen pain that you may already have.

324.    If you are deficient in vitamin B-12, you may be at risk for back pain. Studies show that this vitamin can alleviate low back pain. People who receive vitamin B-12 injections, show a statistically significant reduction in pain and disability. Meat and dairy products are some other good ways to get vitamin B-12.

325.    A lot of people who do not sleep on a regular schedule experience back pain, so try to get at least seven hours of sleep per night on a regular schedule. Staying awake and on your feet for prolonged hours puts a lot of stress on your back and can ultimately result in moderate to severe pain. Sleeping will help decrease this.

326.    One of the best ways to ease your back pain is to flip. Flip your mattress. The springs and inner build up of your mattress can settle over time. Turn your mattress clockwise. Next time, flip it completely over. By doing this it will help your mattress wear evenly which will ease your pain.

327.    The best time to stretch your muscles to help eliminate back pain is while your muscles are still

warm. Always stretch as part of your cool-down routine after exercising.

328.   For people who experience chronic back pain, your first visit shouldn't be to the store to purchase a massager but rather to the doctor's office to see if you have a slipped disc or another type of injury. Back pain can be the result of a hundred different things, and many of them can be serious.

329.   Sleeping in a good position that works for your body will help to reduce straining of your back at night. Use your comfort to be your guide, and don't try to sleep in a certain position because you heard it was the right thing to do. Everybody is different, and will have different needs.

330.   A way to decrease back pain that is not often considered is to raise the size of your fonts on your computer. The logic is simple: if you can't read something on your computer screen, you tend to hunch over your computer to read it. By increasing your font size, you alleviate the need to hunch over and, therefore, decrease the strain on your back!